RELUCTANT HEALER

An Introduction to Energy Healing

Susana Stoica, Ph.D.

The intent of this book is to provide a better understanding of energy medicine, not to promote it to the exclusion of allopathic medicine. To the contrary, I know from my own experience that using both mainstream medical methods and alternative medical solutions can improve the current treatment spectrum and offer solutions where none are known today.

ISBN-13: 978-0965457538

ISBN-10: 0965457532

Healing Alternatives
Press
P.O. Box 3263
Farmington Hills
MI 48333, U.S.A.

I started gradually having problems with my field of vision. By the time I got to the eye doctor I was seeing mainly on the periphery of my visual field. I was told that the visual nerve in my left eye was dying off and was sent to an eye neurologist without being given any kind of hope of recovery—maybe just a slim chance of stopping the progress. At this point, I contacted Susana Stoica, who immediately started doing healing sessions via Skype. Because I lived alone, I could not provide her with the pictures she requested for long-distance healing. After the first session, I started to see somewhat better. After the third session, I completely regained my vision. By the time I got to the eye neurologist my nerve was completely healed! Thank you, Susana!

Ann Wagenberg, 71 years old, Tel Aviv, Israel

We struggled with unexplained infertility for approximately ten years. After going through four rounds of IVF treatments, which failed, we decided to try the holistic approach, which led us to Susana Stoica. Susana's energy healing/balancing was able to release stored stress and anxiety that was affecting our ability to conceive. With Susana's help we now have three beautiful, healthy children of our own. We continue to use Susana's gifts of healing when we recognize our bodies are sluggish, out of sync, and in need of balancing. After the sessions we always feel energized, rested, and focused.

Dave & Rhonda, Farmington Hills, Michigan, USA

I first met Susana in the early nineties when I had pancreatitis following gall bladder surgery. Susana came to the hospital and [with the doctor's permission] did Healing Touch on me. To the doctor's surprise, a hospital stay that should have lasted ten days was shortened to two days! More recently, Susana did some healing on my knee, which was damaged in a fall about fifteen years ago, and my hip, which was injured a few years ago. The injury to my knee made walking difficult and affected my gait, and the hip injury made walking even more difficult. During the session I felt my whole body tingling as if stars were shooting through it. Almost instantly the pain in my knee was gone, which allowed me to begin moving without wobbling. An additional side effect of the session was a feeling of peace and well-being. Thanks Susana! What an amazing gift you have!

Nicole Hartrell, Toronto, Canada

I was feeling very sick for about two weeks with bloating, stomach spasms, loss of appetite, hot/cold flushes, and a total lack of energy (I couldn't even walk my dog), so I finally contacted Susana Stoica. She immediately told me I had a virus and recommended a very simple home remedy, telling me that she would work on me the next day. By the next morning I felt a big improvement. I no longer had the nausea and dizziness I had wakened with each morning for the past two weeks! After Susana worked on me the virus was gone. It was like a switch had been turned on in my body! By the end of that day I felt incredible, and by the next day it was like I had never been sick. I haven't looked back since. AMAZING! I just wish I had called her sooner!

Sue Sieber, Phoenix, Arizona, USA

My wife contacted Susana for energy healing to repair the neural damage caused by successive unsuccessful fertility treatments. At the end of what could be offered by modern medicine, we had given up hope that we could have a child of our own. When it was my turn to enter the healing process, Susana told me that one day we would have that child we wanted so much. A little more than nine months later, our son, Kyle, arrived to brighten our lives, followed by a brother two years later. Only those who have shared the pain of not being able to have children can understand the gift that Susana's special talent has brought to our lives.

Bruce Hulscher, D.D.S.
Michigan Institute of Advanced Dentistry, Michigan, USA

I was diagnosed with cancer for the fourth time in September 2008. I knew even before being diagnosed again that I had some strong emotional issues from my teenage years that I needed to deal with, but

I hadn't come across the right venue to help me access them. I was introduced to Susana by my sister shortly after my last diagnosis, and what a blessing! Susana's gifts of energy healing and Journey sessions allowed me to uncover, address, and release those negative emotions and energies that were affecting my health. With Susana's help, I am now healthy and have more energy, clarity, and overall wellbeing. Her many insights gave me the confidence to trust myself and the ability to continue my journey toward achieving optimum health.

Sarah Iverson, Minneapolis, Minnesota, USA

Other books by the same author:

Heal Your Brain, Reclaim Your Life: How to Recover and Thrive after a Concussion

Cooking after Brain Injury: Easy Cooking for Recovery – Books 1 - 5

Five Mirrors, Five Blessings

Healing with the Loving Heart

To my father, who taught me never to be afraid to go into uncharted territories of human knowledge, and to my son, Andrei, so that he may do the same.

Contents

Introduction to the Second Edition

Many years have passed since I first wrote this book. My life has changed in a lot of ways since then. I experienced a traumatic brain injury and I was incapable of doing any kind of healing work for some time, while at the same time my medical intuition was many times better as I no longer had the "filter" normally provided by my frontal brain to hold me back. My knowledge as a healer helped me limit the effects of the head injury and provided solutions where traditional medical science had nothing to offer. The experience made me more compassionate as well as more knowledgeable as a healer.

Rereading the book from this new vantage point was an interesting experience. In a way it felt like I was reading somebody else's story, while the story of my struggle to accept myself as a healer helped me rally once again and restart my life. I remembered my father's passion for helping people and the pleasure both he and I had doing it. I also knew that the "new me" had something valuable to offer: my experience of successfully using what I knew about healing to recover from my own brain injury.

It was especially interesting to read the second part of the book in which I answered some questions about healing. I realized how much more knowledge and experience I had since first writing the book. As a result, I decided to update that part with some interesting insights and to add some simple examples for perceiving and working with the human energy field.

I hope my story will give others the necessary willpower to go on and search for solutions for their own healing when mainstream medical knowledge has nothing more to offer.

I am interested to hear your feedback on the book and to answer any questions you might have. You can reach me via email at: **healingbraininjury@gmail.com**.

Foreword

I am excited to work with *The Reluctant Healer*. My practice incorporates Western medicine as well as acupuncture and other natural therapies. I feel that all of us, whether medical doctors or healers, work in an energetic model as described in this book, even if we don't realize it.

The Reluctant Healer is a wonderful story about a healer recognizing her powers and utilizing them to help others. Susana accurately describes how one's energy field can influence health and illness. I frequently see patients who complain of "having no energy," but I was not trained in medical school how to evaluate such a statement.

My study of acupuncture involved learning about energy meridians, and I was very interested to find that Susana's description of balancing one's energy field coincides with the meridian-balancing theories in acupuncture. I know from my practice that the balancing of one's bio-energy flow is a prerequisite to good health. *The Reluctant Healer* describes Susana's search for channeling this energy flow to achieve a healthy state.

The book describes twenty-first-century energy medicine. Once all patients and doctors alike learn to look at all illness and health in an energetic model, medicine will leap forward.

As Susana's book tells the story of her journey of searching and using this energetic model to treat patients, I hope it will be of help to both patients and doctors who want to understand the energetic model of maintaining one's health.

David Brownstein, MD
Detroit, Michigan
1996

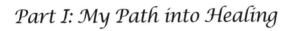

Part I: My Path into Healing

There is nothing more frustrating than watching a loved one suffer and struggle with illness. At first the person cannot eat certain foods or move in certain ways. Next discomfort starts to affect concentration. If the condition is not successfully treated, the person's entire way of life is affected. The outward signs of an illness are both clear and unpleasant, but the causes are often mysterious, making treatment extremely difficult.

At the beginning of my path into healing, I had no formal training in understanding these causes, yet felt compelled to act, to change something, to fight the pain in some way. Like most people, I took my family members to see a medical professional when they became ill, trusting that the medical professional would offer a definite, scientific cure. The doctor first had to determine which one of a number of potential illnesses could be causing those particular symptoms. Often, in more critical situations, the doctor tried different medications until one eventually seemed to work. My loved one started to feel like the object of an experiment. In the end, he might not even have been able to take the best available medication because of allergies.

Disappointed with traditional medical approaches, I began giving my family members simple herbal remedies that I knew from childhood. To my surprise and delight, those herbal remedies helped where sophisticated drugs did not. Encouraged by these early attempts and motivated by a strong internal desire to help, I tried to find alternative solutions to other illnesses. Eventually, I found myself in the middle of completely uncharted territory where my previous training was of no guidance and in situations for which I had no explanation.

This book is about my personal experiences related to energy medicine, something we call *healing*. While medical doctors are themselves healers, the term *healer* in this book is used to describe people who are practicing energy medicine.

The first part of the book alternates between chapters relating the story of my journey into healing and the event that caused me to write it—my father's cancer surgery. The second part of the book presents my views on healing in the context of real-life experiences and answers questions I am commonly asked about healing.

I trust that my professional standing will dispel the traditional view of the healer as an esoteric person with his/her head in the clouds. From what I have seen, true healers do not practice their skill because they choose to, but because they feel they must help others. They take their work very seriously and, as any other professional, are continuously expanding their skills.

I know from personal experience that being a healer is

not a simple endeavor. In the beginning, each one of us is faced with unusual experiences, and many times we do not know how to make sense of them. Unless one has a family member knowledgeable in the field, it takes a while to figure out how to categorize our experiences and thus be able to find a mentor to direct us. As such, I hope this book will show those starting in the healing profession that they are not alone, that others experienced the same doubts and difficulties, and that no one has all the answers.

I also encourage medical doctors to read this book with an open mind and to try using energy medicine as an adjunct to their current medical practice. Doing so would offer patients a broader spectrum of solutions to their health problems. Having worked in a medical practice, I have personally seen the wonderful results of the collaboration between healers and doctors.

The First Day

Following a bad cold in December 1994, my father had an X-ray that showed changes in the texture of the upper right area of his lung. Due to the positioning of the growth, a subsequent biopsy reached close to but not quite the middle of the affected area. The result showed no dangerous cell formations. A later MRI[1] showed that there was still something there, and a follow-up biopsy confirmed the presence of large-cell cancer.[2] He was immediately scheduled for surgery.

After surgery, Dad's recovery was quite normal for the first few days. Even so, by Friday of that week I had a feeling that my father was in some kind of trouble and I had to be with him. When I have such feelings, they usually prove to be true, so on Saturday morning I took the first flight to New York.

I was very anxious to get to the hospital, and when I finally arrived, I found my father very weak, pleading with the nurses not to force him to get out of bed.

---

[1] *MRI*—Magnetic Resonance Imaging—is an imaging method that enables doctors to see structures inside the body

[2] Large-cell cancer is considered less likely to spread.

Apparently, a nurse had forced him to get out of bed the previous night, and something happened that made him feel much worse. His appearance and behavior concerned me, as it was quite unusual for him to want to stay in bed.

Dad's familiar warm but determined face was quite pale, and he was obviously drained of energy. Despite his nearly seventy-seven years, Dad normally looked and behaved like a man of fifty-five at most. During the day he was always on the move: repairing things, helping family and friends, doing things around the house, or learning new things. He was the kind of man who could not sit on the sidelines when he saw a problem. For him, there was always something that could be done to improve a critical situation—but this case was different. He was desperately trying to control the situation, and it was extremely unnerving for him that he could not. His own body was proving to be his biggest challenge.

Like a typical engineer, Dad was trying to determine for himself what was going on and was monitoring his own medical "parameters." He was feeling more and more let down by the setback and the lack of explanation for the source of the problem. His condition was only getting worse due to his impatience. I was wishing I was a medical doctor so I could help him, or so I could at least explain the complicated medical jargon used by the doctors. He wanted to be an active participant in his healing process, but there was no obvious way in which he could do so.

The first day I arrived passed as a regular hospital day: visits, tests, treatments. We were watching Dad get more and more tired, but our presence was obviously comforting him. I volunteered to spend the night at the hospital, letting my sister take a well-deserved rest.

As Saturday night progressed, the situation became increasingly critical. Dad's lungs constantly filled with phlegm, creating problems with his breathing. The nurses were in and out of the room all night trying to suction his lungs, pounding and massaging his back, and turning him from one side to another, but nothing they did helped for long. After about half an hour, his lungs once again filled with phlegm.

By two o'clock in the morning the nurses told me they could not do much more. Despite their best efforts, they could no longer remove the phlegm that kept accumulating.

The Big Decision

As do all other healers, I work with the human energy field, also known as the *aura*. The aura penetrates the whole physical body and extends outside it. It can be felt as a very fine vibration of even frequency all around the healthy body. Some healers can see the aura as an array of colors superimposed over the physical body.

The meaning of aura colors varies from one healer to another, but generally the clearer colors are considered healthy, while the darker, dirty-looking ones are signs of possible problems. After their first healing session, people often say that they perceive the colors in their environment as more vibrant. This is because we see through our aura. When we are sick, the aura becomes darker and murkier, putting a dirty "window" between us and our environment. Once the aura is cleaned, we can see the real colors around us. I assume this is the reason why sick people often tend to have a "darker" outlook on life, while healthy individuals are usually happier.

In a healthy person, the aura has certain regions that appear as rotating cones. These are the energy centers of the aura, also known as *chakras*. The chakras act as the communication channels between the energy field and the environment. If they are partially or totally closed or damaged in any way, the energy field gets blocked, and sickness occurs in the physical body. To maintain the health of the aura, the energy centers must be fully open and functioning normally. If the aura is already damaged in any way (torn, blocked, or stuffed with unusual accumulations of energy, for example), the chakras tend to be overstressed and eventually damaged. Hence, the damaged areas of the aura and the chakras must be cleaned and repaired before the person can recover. *The energy field is like the mold for the physical body.* If the mold is damaged, what it holds—in other words, the physical body—is also damaged.

While to an average observer it may seem that a healer works in a random pattern, this is far from accurate. The methods might vary, but every healer first visually or manually scans the aura for energy irregularities, evaluating the extent of the damage and the order in which the damaged regions must be approached. Once the energy disturbances are located, the healer uses his or her preferred methods to clean, repair, and re-pattern the energy field until it has an even structure all over. Unfortunately, because of the wide variety of available methodologies and the impossibility exactly predicting the results, healing meets with resistance and misunderstanding.

That March night in the hospital, alone with my

exhausted father—my dad, my friend, my mentor—I was thinking of how powerless one is when faced with these types of crises. My heart was breaking as I watched his breathing become more and more labored. I thought I had no power to help him. I was being held back by a promise I was forced to make to my family before being allowed to come and stay with Dad: that I would not do "that stuff"—in other words, I would not practice healing on him.

Due to repeated medical interventions, my father was very tired. Even fighting for every breath could not wake him. The phlegm kept accumulating in his lungs, and I could see he would soon choke. Many thoughts were racing through my mind: *What am I going to do? I could probably help him, but my family made me promise not to use healing! I helped so many people before, why not Dad? What if they are right and my treatment interferes with the medication? What about my promise? I have never broken a promise, but I have to if I want to help him.*

I thought of the strong feeling that drove me to the hospital, how much my father had done for us all his life, how much he meant to us, and how many people I helped before with my healing (with none of them having any negative reactions). I tried to relax and think of the options available for him. Suddenly Dad's breath was so labored that I felt he would soon choke to death unless I did something about it. It was a choice between doing what I did so many times before or keeping my word and possibly risking his life. I did not want to harm him, but the nurses told me that there was nothing more they could do. I did not want to keep him from something that had helped so many others, so I decided to start working on Dad.

Immediately my hands assumed a life of their own, flying over my father's body. I no longer hesitated. While scanning his aura, I could feel his collapsed energy centers. The energy over his lungs was thick and vibrating slower than over the rest of his body. The area of the surgery presented a disruption in the field, which is usually perceived as missing energy. The energy in his lower abdomen felt like thick mud. I could find very little energy in his legs. The lack of energy in his legs was a dangerous sign, as people who are gravely ill or ready to depart usually first lose the energy in their legs. This finding made me even more worried, but I knew too well that I had to be completely relaxed and objective if I wanted to do the healing.

First, I cleaned the energy field, removing the slow energy from the lung area. It was best not to work on my father for very long, as he was too weak. It would have been too sudden a shock for his system. After about ten minutes, I was relieved to see his breathing calm down a little, and I took a break. I repeated the treatment two more times at half-hour intervals until I felt he was out of danger. Then I dropped off to sleep.

We both slept peacefully until six in the morning when the night nurses started coming in for their regular morning rounds. Looking at the charts, they realized we had not called for help after two o'clock. They were surprised to see my father, who had slept so calmly, with more color in his face. They started asking what happened, but I knew it would be foolish to tell them the truth. Since the medical staff easily accepted sudden remissions, I simply told them that he suddenly calmed down. This worked with all the nurses except one. She was too dedicated to her patients to let the matter go so easily. Reluctantly, and carefully testing her level of acceptance, I told her the real story. To my surprise, she was very understanding—she knew a nurse on another floor who studied Therapeutic Touch[3] and who was applying it from time to time. (I was doing Healing Touch, which is also an energy healing method taught in nursing schools.[4])

Unfortunately, working on my father during the day was out of the question. I had to wait until the next night to continue. This gave me plenty of time to think over the events of the previous night and how I arrived at what I was doing.

---

[3] Therapeutic Touch is an energy healing method developed and championed by Dolores Krieger and Dora Kunz. It is taught at nursing schools and to lay people.

[4] Healing Touch is an energy healing method developed and championed by Janet Mentgen. It combines a number of healing modalities and is taught worldwide both to nurses and to lay practitioners.

The Early Years

While my father was resting, my thoughts went back to my first experience with healing. I was about seven.

My sister was very sickly as a baby. She had infections all the time in her ears, adenoids, and throat. The doctor had to come to our home so frequently that my parents decided to pay him by the month to make sure he was available when we needed him. My sister cried nearly every night. I could see my parents becoming more and more tired as the weeks passed. I offered to take care of my sister for one night, but they were reluctant, since I wasn't even seven years old. I felt very bad about their lack of trust. Finally, my parents relented on the condition that I would wake them if anything happened.

My sister didn't cry at all that night, and we all slept through the night. My mother found us both sleeping in my bed the next morning. Thinking back to my sister's behavior that night, I could equate it to recent times when my sensitive friends like to be in my energy field because they say it is comforting to them. The solid night's sleep might have indicated a similar effect.

I also remember a time when my mother split her forehead open on a window pane that happened to be in her way as she hurried to work. Blood was gushing from the cut so badly that we had to call for an ambulance. My father, who was our "emergency family doctor," usually fainted at the sight of blood, so he called on me to help. He explained what had to be done and let me do it. I was pretty much on my own, and I was proud Dad trusted me.

While waiting for the ambulance to arrive, I remember cleaning the wound and putting the sides of the cut back together. I went over the cut with my finger several times, wishing I could seal it. Then I bandaged Mom's forehead the best I knew how. By the time the ambulance came, my mother was cleaned and bandaged. The bandage was quite large, but my father was happy that the bandage was in place and he couldn't see any bleeding. With that, he could help comfort Mother.

The ambulance took both of my parents to the hospital. When the doctor removed the bandage, there was no bleeding and no need for the customary stitches. He recommended that whoever did the original bandaging should continue to do so from now on, changing the bandages at regular intervals. Mom went for a checkup later and everything was in order. The wound healed without a scar.

After my first experience as a healer, I learned the rest of the story from my father. The doctor who saw my mother at the hospital asked who did such a good job on the wound, and my father proudly told him, "It was my seven-year-old daughter." My father was smiling like a Cheshire cat when he arrived home, still having fun remembering the doctor's puzzled reaction!

I did not think too much about the incident at the time. Like any other kid would be, I was happy Mom was back home and not bleeding. After all, my father had done all sorts of similar things for us when we were sick, so it seemed perfectly normal for me to help at the time.

With the passage of years, I found myself observing my father as he took emergency measures when we were ill. He had a special intuition for what to do when we were not feeling well and had to wait until morning to call a doctor. Later, I ended up trying to guess what he was going to "prescribe": aspirin, alcohol rubdown, hot tea with honey, or herbal teas. His repertoire was not large, but we always felt better after his "cure."

The years passed; I got married and had a son. As with every child, he had his share of problems, from ear infections to scarlet fever. I remember that every time we went to the pediatrician, as soon as we stepped into her office, she asked me the same two questions: "What do you think your son has?" and "What did you give him?" She always enjoyed it if I provided the right "diagnosis" and medication. She usually told me to follow the same treatment I had already started. I never thought about this as being out of the ordinary, since my father had a real talent for correctly diagnosing our illnesses.

The Second Night

Suddenly my thoughts shifted back to the present.

Sunday night I had to wait until the nurses were finished with their evening rounds and my father was asleep before I could work on him again. He was still having problems breathing when he stayed on his back for an extended time. Despite the massaging and pounding done by the nurses during the day and a few times during the night, the phlegm kept accumulating.

Finally, once everything became quiet, I was ready for my turn. This time I did not hesitate at all. I could see that while he was still very sick, my father was definitely feeling better than he had the previous night.

First I checked his energy field. I could still feel the disruption due to the surgery as well as the thicker feeling in the lung area. The energy centers were more active but were still collapsed compared to a normal field, which meant that the body could not get proper nourishment from the energetic environment. This made Dad's energy field weaker than normal. The muddy feeling in his abdomen was still there. My focus at that moment was on helping him breathe and become stronger without overtaxing his body, so the work on his abdominal area had to be postponed.

It is known that doctors have a hard time treating their own families, since it is difficult to remain objective. That's even more difficult for healers. One not only has to remain objective but must be very calm and focused during the session, undisturbed by any kind of emotion. Since a healer uses his/her own field as a conduit for healing, emotions can act as energetic noises that, if not controlled, can easily shut off the flow of healing energy. The healer must also adjust his or her own energy field to different energy frequencies during the session in order to deal with the different field disturbances. If one is not completely detached, the ability to sense the different energetic conditions diminishes.

After some experience, I was able to switch off the world around me while I worked. The person I was working on became for me an energy field, and I was able to clearly detect all the physical and emotional level imbalances. Once I was able to master this state of mind, the healing sessions became much more effective, and I was able to deal with the whole healing process in a much clearer and more objective manner. With time, I was even able to talk to the person I was working with while staying focused on changes in the energy field.[5]

---

[5] These days I do virtually all my healing work from a distance because I concentrate even better, making my work more effective.

That Sunday night I started the healing session by quieting down and lightly balancing[6] the field. I followed this by removing congestion in the lung area from the field[7] and raising and strengthening the energy centers. Since my father was still weak, I had to keep my own field frequency and amplitude relatively low.

My father's breathing responded well. His breathing soon became much calmer and more even but, unfortunately, it was still not normal. I also directed energy into the site of the surgery to repair the damage to the energy field and aid the wound's healing process.[8] Next, I performed a gentle balancing of the overall field[9] using the palms of my hands to interconnect different areas of the body and reestablish a correct energy flow.

---

[6] Balancing is done by letting one's hand go over the whole energetic body with a smoothing motion, gently connecting the energy field centers.

[7] Congestion is removed by moving through the energetic field with the fingers acting as combs capable of catching the unwanted energetic accumulations.

[8] The techniques used are known as "modulating energy" into the wounded area. They are used for replenishing the energy lost due to the field disruption. "Lasering" the field is then used to close the energy wound. These two techniques are known to be quite effective in accelerating the healing of all sorts of wounds and energy breaks. The first one is performed by directing energy through the healer's palms into the person's energetic body. Lasering is done by using one's fingers like laser heads. As the energy is more focused at the tip of one's fingers, the effect of this technique over the energetic body is very similar to the effect of the laser on the physical body.

[9] This technique is known in Healing Touch as the "full body connection" at etheric level.

At the end, I closed all the layers of the energy field[10] to prevent the energy that was directed into his field from escaping. To do this, I let my palms walk over the full length of his field in a continuous motion while willing to enclose him in an egg-shaped form of light.

Since Dad was breathing easier, the night was more peaceful than the previous one. Unfortunately, the test results the next morning showed that his blood count was dangerously low. The doctors decided to strengthen my father by giving him a transfusion of four pints of blood.

The rest of the day's events were made up of the normal hospital routine while I waited for the night so I could continue my work. In the meantime, yet again, I was thinking about my path into healing.

---

[10] The closing of the field is necessary to make sure that the effects of the healing session are lasting. This is especially important when treating people who are very sick or extremely tired and who are typically losing energy.

Searching for a Cure

My path into healing work emerged over the years with many starts and stops. The first major step was prompted by my husband's recurring back pains. He was confined to bed several times a year, but there was not much that could be done, especially since he did not like to go to the doctor. Being used to acting as the "emergency family doctor" since childhood, I decided to do something about it. As a researcher, my life was dedicated to studying. It seemed only logical that I should be able to find a book to help him. Sure enough, after attending a presentation on Reflexology[11] in 1981, I bought several books and studied them on my own.

I had always been curious and intrigued by the human nervous system[12] and its reaction to external stimuli, so I

---

[11] Reflexology is the study of reflexes in the feet, hands, and ears that correspond to all other areas of the body. It is based on the zone theory developed by Dr. William Fitzgerald in the early 1900s. The most popular is foot reflexology. The practitioner of this method applies deep massage to eliminate the sandy deposits from the zones corresponding to the affected areas. The method is less intrusive than acupuncture, and those who have the experience and sensitivity to find the points can relieve a host of physical complaints.

[12] This eventually brought me to study the electronic circuits that model the

was very interested in studying Reflexology. I learned and memorized all the different regions of the hands and feet, and I could reference the body regions represented in the ears. Unfortunately, once I mastered the treatment method, I was surprised to find out that I could not utilize it on my "healing target"—my husband's feet were much too sensitive.

Not being easily discouraged, I continued my search. One day, while looking for a professional book at Canada's largest bookstore, I stopped at the medical section. I was looking for something that offered a non-intrusive method of treatment and did not require any strong action on the individual. I soon found a book that presented the Polarity[13] treatment, a form of treatment that requires only a gentle touching of the person. I started paging through the book with excitement—it was exactly what I needed.

I studied the book very carefully, set up diagrams of the treatments, and plastered them on the wall. I was ready to try working on my husband again. Then I noticed that

---

nervous system behavior, known as threshold logic gates, and later as neural nets. I ended up writing both my M.Sc. and Ph.D. theses on this subject.

[13] Polarity, inspired by traditional Chinese medicine, was created by Dr. Randolph Stone. It defines the human body as a polarized energy field. During the session the practitioner acts as a connector between the positive and negative sides of the person's energy field with the intent of restoring the overall balance necessary for good health.

there was a strong warning in the book: Do not use the treatments unless properly trained, as one can get some unexpected results—like sudden outbursts of anger. Now I had a problem: how could I find a teacher who could give me the proper training?

In the meantime, my son became very ill. He was having strong stomach pains and had to stay home from school at least one or two days each week. I could see that he was genuinely suffering: he would get very pale and start sweating. Finally, the doctor gave him an antibiotic that made him feel somewhat better for the first three days but then caused him to become much worse. The doctor next prescribed three other medications to fix the damage done by the first one and gave us a very gloomy prediction: my son would suffer from stomachache episodes for at least another eight years due to a "weak stomach lining."

I was shattered. I did not want my son to be practically crippled until he turned eighteen. I could see him having to go through the same pain again and again, needing more and more medication and not being able to enjoy what should have been the most carefree years of his life. I went home without filling the prescription and decided to think it over. It occurred to me that people had used all sorts of teas, soups, and baths before over-the-counter medicines were available. In fact, everybody used to have them at home. I knew that medicine contained only the active ingredients from plants, which were artificially reproduced in the labs. In the process, we were losing the overall effect of the herb. By the next morning I made my decision: I was going to try to find an herbal remedy before getting my son on a roller coaster of medications.

I was once again in the medical section of Toronto's largest bookstore when I easily found an herbal reference book. I studied the book that night, and by morning I had the right herbal combination for my son. There was only one problem: the tea that I decided to give him contained herbs not usually available in health-food stores. After a few false starts, I found a very a good herbal store run by a kind and very knowledgeable owner. He helped me understand the correct measurement and preparation of the different teas from roots, leaves, and flowers. A few days after starting to drink the tea, my son was better. Within a month he was in perfect health. Three weeks later, he started feeling a slight stomach pain. After he drank the same tea for another week, his complaints never returned. It had been only two months—far from the *eight years* the doctor predicted.

Unfortunately, the solution for my husband's back pain was not that easy, but my visit to the herb store proved instrumental in finding ways to help him. That visit opened unexpected opportunities for following my path into healing.

The Third Day

My thoughts, which had drifted to Reflexology, Polarity, and herbs, returned to the task at hand. It was Monday morning, and the doctors were really concerned about my father's blood count. They decided to give Dad another two pints of blood. His breathing was better, so my concern shifted to the muddy feeling in his abdomen, which by now I could relate to the internal bleeding diagnosed by the doctors.

By this time, I felt too tired to continue the energy healing sessions at night. Fortunately, my father was a bit better, so I asked his permission to work on him during the day. We had a lengthy discussion, since he did not believe in "the stuff" I was doing. I decided to speak his language: engineering reasoning. If "the stuff" did not do anything, there was nothing to be concerned about. However, if it *did* do something, I assured him, the only risk was feeling better. I told him about cases I worked with, and he asked many questions. Dad still did not believe in what I was doing, but he accepted my argument, so I started working on him during the day.

His energy field felt much better. The disruption in the surgery area was nearly gone. The lung area felt better, although I could still feel some thickness. The chakras started holding the treatment instead of collapsing. I worked mainly on the muddy feeling in the colon[14] area where there were three obvious energy breakage spots; these kinds of breakage usually correspond to wounds. The doctor ordered an upper gastrointestinal X-ray to determine the source of bleeding. Before going to have the X-ray done, my father asked my opinion about whether he should go for the test. I told him they were not going to see anything on the X-ray as they were not going to check the colon area, but at the same time I encouraged him to verify my findings with medical tests. As expected, the X-ray did not find any open wounds.

By now I was working on my father several times a day. When we were alone at night I slept beside him in a chair. It was a real relief to see him being able to breathe and smile again. My mind was much more at ease and once again drifted to my earlier experiences.

---

[14] The colon, also known as the large intestine, is located in the abdominal cavity and consists of the *ascending colon,* the *transverse colon,* and the *descending colon.*

"When the Student Is Ready, the Teacher Will Appear"

I have heard the above saying many times, but I never understood it until the day I went to buy herbs for my son's stomach problem. On the wall of the herbal store was an announcement for a course on Polarity treatments presented by a yoga teacher. I promptly registered for the course.

There I was, waiting for the course that was going to change my life more profoundly than I could ever imagine at the time.

The teacher was well-informed and patient, teaching with the obvious pleasure of a person handing over an enchanted piece of knowledge. He was right: helping somebody's healing process through nothing more than gentle touch was truly something to look forward to. He explained the different hand positions for treatment, and we practiced them on each other. The whole class created a feeling of community between people with the same interest—helping others. We continued the study and practice. At the end of the course the teacher let us go with an interesting bit of advice: "Remember what you are going to dream tonight; it might be interesting."

I went home full of energy and excitement. That night I quickly fell asleep and had two interesting dreams. In the first I saw my body, made completely of light, lying on a massage table. In my physical form, I was working on it. My body on the table was made of a very pleasant, brightly shimmering, white light that I had never seen before. I enjoyed my dream. It gave me a very peaceful feeling and made me feel weightless for some reason. At the same time, I was baffled. By morning I still remembered every detail of the dream, which was quite unusual for me.

In the morning while I was still in a state between dreaming and lucidity, I had a much more interesting dream. I suddenly found myself in a very brightly colored meadow. Everything had that special, bright, shimmering quality from the previous dream, including my light body. I was walking around and got to an area with slightly rolling hills covered with green grass as far as I could see. It was very nice and peaceful. Then a figure made entirely of the same shimmering light appeared from behind a mound and came toward me. He wore a flowing garb that had the same shiny white texture as my body in the previous dream. Over the white garb he wore a sky-blue garb that covered only his front and back. It too seemed to be made of light. His face was very calm. As he came closer, I felt the need to kneel and hold out my hands. The reaction was quite unusual for somebody who considered herself a non-religious, exact scientist. The figure continued walking toward me. Suddenly I could see a large ball of golden light in his hands. When he was right in front of me, he placed the ball in my hands, looking at me as if I knew what to do with it. Then he proceeded to continue his walk by going right through me. I woke up with a jolt, having a sense of deep internal peace yet also overwhelmed by what I had just experienced.

I knew I could not say anything about the dreams to those closest to me, since it would scare them. Anyway, what would I tell them? How could I explain these dreams? I decided the only person who could make sense of all this was my Polarity teacher. But when I told him about the dreams the next morning, he asked, "What do you think it was? You will have to find out for yourself."

Something else happened in class the very next day that made matters even more unsettling. We were told that, to avoid jarring the person's energy field, we should lift our hands slowly when finished with the session. During the morning exercise I proceeded to do just that while working on my partner. Suddenly, to my dismay, my hands just went to the person's lung area, as if attracted by a strong magnet. They started moving very quickly and were out of control. I was quite surprised and shocked. I did not understand what was happening. It did not fit into my frame of knowledge as an engineer, and it was not anything I had experienced or heard of before. I was really baffled and scared, but I could do nothing about it. There seemed to be a gentle but firm force holding my hands in place. I had no control over the furious movement of my hands or where they were going.

My teacher was watching me from the front of the class, and he signaled me to calm down and continue what I was doing. I did not have a choice, so I did just that. Suddenly, in my mind's eye I saw a dark, gray cloud lifting from my partner's lung and coming toward me. By instinct I threw white light (the same kind I saw in my dreams the night before) over the gray cloud, and it disappeared. Then I saw myself inside an old church with a very high ceiling and large stained-glass windows. The sun was coming in, creating a deeply peaceful feeling. I could nearly hear the organ music playing in the church. I tried to analyze what was going on using my usual inquisitiveness, but there was no way I could find any explanation for it.

After a while, which seemed to me like an eternity, my hands stopped, and I could see the whole classroom staring at me. In response to my bewilderment, my teacher said the same things he said that morning: "What do *you* think it was? *You* will have to find out for yourself." This obviously was not too helpful.

We stopped for lunch. I was very quiet and hardly touched the food, as I was quite shaken. At the end of the lunch my partner told the group that she had a bad flu more than a month earlier and had been left with something in her lungs that no one could diagnose or cure, despite all the tests and medication given by various doctors. Now, for the first time in more than a month, she could breathe freely. She thanked me profusely.

I was stunned. I found myself confronted by an exotic and powerful phenomenon with no framework of experience in which I could fit it. I had no idea where it came from, what it was, how it happened, how I could repeat it, whether it worked on anyone at any time, and whether it always worked in the same way. I had thousands of questions in my mind, all unanswered, as I faced this different reality.

To make matters even more complicated, while climbing the stairs to the classroom on our way back from lunch, my partner told me in a quiet voice, "I don't know how to tell you, but. . . ." She then described the same church image that I saw in my mind's eye while working on her. That really shook me up!

We finished the course and I went home dazed. I did not understand what happened, my teacher was of no help, and my logical mind was constantly fighting between accepting and discarding all that happened that day. I was partly curious, partly overwhelmed, and a good amount scared.

I went home bursting to tell my husband, but as soon as I started telling him, his response was, "You can do whatever you choose to, but don't tell me about it." I understood that I was completely alone in a pursuit unlike any other I had attempted in my life. When I wanted to explore a new field before, I went to the library. This time, I could not put any label on my experiences and had no starting point for my research.

For several days I pondered what to do. The next week I went back to the yoga center where we had the course so I could take part in the weekly meditation session. It only brought back that "certain feeling" but didn't bring me any closer to an explanation.

In the hope that I would gain some understanding, I went to a more detailed course on Elemental Polarity that was taught by the same person. He taught us the Hindu Ayurvedic medicine method of balancing the three elements in the body, known as *vata*, *pitta*, and *kapha*, but he was teaching it using the five elements accepted by Western esoteric tradition: earth, water, fire, air, and ether.

The course was very interesting, but I had a problem with it: the method required the healer to push inside the body for the heavier elements, starting from earth, and then use a progressively lighter touch going toward the lighter elements. Despite all my best efforts to do the practice correctly, an invisible hand seemed to be pushing my hand out of the body and above it. I was quite upset. I wanted to do the exercises as they were taught, but I could not. I had studied many things in my life and I was always able to repeat the things I was taught. Not this time. Finally, I approached the teacher, who simply told me, "If this is what is happening, this is what you are meant to do." Unfortunately, he did not tell me what *this* was!

During the following two years I read all sorts of books about alternative medicine, Leadbetter's works [9] about Edgar Cayce [4, 7], and Kilner's classic [8] on human energy fields. I finally had a name for what I was doing — *healing*— but I still had no explanation that could stand up to scientific standards.

The Fourth Day

My thoughts came back to the hospital room and to my father. He was still weak, but his breathing had improved considerably. The energy break in the surgery area started to heal and was obviously smaller. The energy centers were not as collapsed as before, so I changed the focus of my healing to his abdominal area.

From an energetic point of view, my father was on his way to healing himself.[15] The energy field felt strong enough that he could withstand a more intense session. I balanced his field, mending and re-patterning the energy in all the damaged areas of the colon. At the end, I energized the entire field and closed it to make sure that the treatment would hold.

I worked on my father several times that day, half an hour at a time, when no one could see us. I still wanted to be with him in the hospital. The pain of his surgery started to subside, and Dad felt less drained. From now

---

[15] The name given to healers is in a way incorrect, as the person doing the healing is merely cleaning, balancing, and strengthening the person's energy field. The change in the person's health status is due to his body's improved capability to fight the illness given by the stronger and healthier energy field.

on I used the evening sessions only for relaxation and did healing sessions during the day.

The best news of the day was that Dad's blood count did not go down for the first time since Saturday, which meant that the bleeding had stopped. However, the doctors still wanted to see where the bleeding was coming from and decided to order a lower gastro-intestinal X-ray for Friday.

Before falling asleep that night, I thought about the tremendous healing power that could be offered to people by combining medical science and energy medicine and how much we could find out about health and illness by using the two techniques together. If only there was some logical explanation for healing, doctors could accept it much easier!

There Is No Logical Answer

Slowly I began to understand that there was no such thing as a logical explanation for what I was doing. It had to be accepted for what it was. Also, I started to understand what our teacher had repeatedly told us during the Polarity course: not to get attached to the results of our healing work. According to his teaching, a healer must be "like an empty flute through which the energy can pass unhindered." It was difficult to understand this because it could not be explained—it had to be experienced.

Like every healer, I had my share of acquired aches and pains until I understood the above lesson. When working with a Parkinson's patient, I temporarily acquired the characteristic lack of mental clarity. When working with people undergoing chemotherapy, I felt extremely nauseated during the session. These phenomena were quite unpleasant, but they usually went away after a good, restful sleep.

I started doing what I thought was Polarity on my family and friends. It always worked for a flu, a headache, or a sprained ankle. I was delighted by the results, and I became less and less uncomfortable. I found myself being able to switch more easily from my engineering reality to the healing reality. Soon I found the two to be quite complementary: engineering provided a more organized approach to healing, while the healing work enhanced my mind's creative side. I found it fascinating that the same mental state was required for creative problem solving and healing. This state can be best defined as relaxed concentration. To be an effective healer, one must be completely relaxed and disconnected from the din of daily events while, at the same time, being focused on the person whose energy field is being worked on. One must concentrate on channeling energy to the correct place and in the correct manner.

Working on close family members became an accepted practice in our home. I remember my husband having a bad ulcer in 1985. It reached the point where Tagamet, the medication prescribed by the doctor, was no longer helping. My husband experienced acute pain during the healing session, but in three days all the ulcer pain was gone. I found that his energy field felt broken with several five-inch (ten- to twelve-centimeter) ridges running vertically in parallel and quite deep in the field above the ulcer. As the ridges became less and less apparent, his ulcer pain started subsiding. During the sessions I also found that he felt less and less of the energy shift as the physical condition of the energy field improved. Before this experience, I was only guessing that this might be the case. Even though there was no logical answer for the sudden remission of the ulcer, our family doctor was very happy that he did not have to take more drastic measures.

One day I noticed that the skin on my son's upper arm exhibited something that looked like stretch marks. He was tired, which could be explained by his very full schedule at school, but that didn't seem to explain the stretch marks, which were becoming more and more apparent. We finally took him to the doctor.

The doctor immediately diagnosed our son as having something wrong with his adrenal glands, a diagnosis confirmed by a twenty-four-hour urine test. He was certain that our son had a tumor of the adrenal gland and sent him for an X-ray. Fortunately, it took about two weeks to schedule the X-ray. This provided me the opportunity to start working on him.

His kidney area felt energetically hot like an electric iron on its highest setting. Not knowing what to expect, I worked on my son every other day, allowing his body time to adapt to the new state of balance. After about ten days the area felt much better; both the structure and the temperature of the field became normal. The X-ray result was "undecided." The doctor was thinking about a biopsy to see what was going on.

By this time the kidney area felt completely normal from an energetic point of view, so I decided to ask the doctor to repeat the original test instead of doing a biopsy. It was tough to give him an acceptable reason, so I decided to tell him the story of what I was doing. He was open-minded and agreed to repeat the urine test, which came back normal. The doctor indicated that such a result just does not usually happen and could not be explained medically. He agreed, however, that if the test was normal there was no reason to go ahead with the biopsy. He repeated the same test two more times. Each time the test result was normal. I continued working on my son for a few more weeks, once or twice a week, and with time the stretch marks became less visible.

I began to feel increasingly more comfortable with healing, yet despite all the good results with my family, I was still uneasy talking about it.

My greatest test came a few years later when I was diagnosed with a fibroid tumor. I felt nauseous every time I tried to do my yoga exercises. Later, I started to feel sick without doing anything out of the ordinary. By the time I went to the doctor, the ultrasound and checkup showed that I had a tumor about the size of a very large grapefruit. The doctor wanted to immediately perform a complete hysterectomy, but I refused. I thought that if I could help others, somebody should be able to help me.

After some time, I found a very good homeopathic

doctor[16] who practiced in the Boston area and with whom I was able to establish a long-distance treatment schedule. Unfortunately, after a few weeks, I had to stop the treatments because they were giving me terrible headaches. Then I noticed that the tumor always grew when I was under stress, so I decided to do everything possible to relax and try healing techniques on myself. I did healing meditations, visualizing white healing light streaming into the tumor. I applied castor oil packs, followed a stringent program of rest, and tried my best not to get upset. Finally, after more than a year, the tumor was reduced to the size of a hazelnut. I was elated. I could again function normally!

Unfortunately, one year later during a time when I was under a lot of stress, the tumor started to grow again. I decided to have it removed. The surgeon said he had never seen such a tumor before: composed entirely of muscle, it was completely unattached to other tissue and "popped out" when the tissue covering it was cut. It had gone from a tumor that was the size of a very large grapefruit and marginally cancerous, according to the homeopathic doctor's tests, to one that was completely benign and the size of a small bird's egg at the time of the surgery!

---

[16] Homeopathy was developed in the eighteenth century by Samuel Hahnemann, a German physician. Homeopathy relies on very small doses of highly diluted remedies to catalyze healing responses.

I was happy and most grateful to be healthy again. This experience gave me a better understanding of suffering and how it affects both the patient and his family. It also gave me the needed incentive to treat my extended family.

*

* *

I was brought back again from my thoughts about healing by the din of the hospital and the constant coming and going of the nursing staff checking on my father.

The Fifth and Sixth Day

On Wednesday my father's blood count started going up for the first time since Saturday. He was breathing easier and was obviously getting stronger. When evaluating his energy field, I could feel three areas damaged by the internal bleeding: the middle of the ascending colon (right-hand side), the transverse colon (liver area), and the lower part of the descending colon (lower left side). The areas were smaller than when I started the healing sessions. The area on the transverse colon was nearly normal again, and the muddy texture of the field had become more fluid. By this time the energy centers started to function more normally and were no longer collapsing. Also, the energy field differences in the surgery wound area were nearly undetectable. By afternoon, my father was on his feet for the first time since Saturday, the first day I had seen him.

The healing sessions that day were aimed at re-patterning the energy in the colon area. This was done by weaving the energy field back to its original structure, sending energy into the surgery area and generally strengthening the field. While I could hardly feel any energy disturbance in the transverse colon, I still directed some energy there to make sure that everything was in the best possible condition. I repeated the sessions several times during the day, making sure at the end of each session that all the layers of the energy field were closed.

On Thursday, the blood tests showed considerable improvement. My father started walking in earnest. Upon testing the energy field, I could still feel some energy residues in the colon area that felt like patches of mud, but nothing as bad as before. Generally, the energy field was much stronger, and the energy centers were all open. The size of the energy centers was smaller than that of a perfectly healthy person, so I worked on them too.

I continued to re-pattern the energy field in the colon area to repair the energetic scars, and I directed energy to the damaged parts. By now, the damage felt much more superficial, and I could work for longer periods of time and more deeply on my father's field. I provided several sessions during the day, and I was happy to see that Dad was walking with more and more confidence as the day unfolded.

The Seventh Day

By Friday, my father's blood count was nearly normal. Checking the energy field in the lower abdomen, I could feel only a minute difference in the field, so slight that it would have been very difficult to detect by somebody who did not know the history of the illness.

The X-ray was scheduled for Friday. Dad was concerned that the doctors would perform another painful procedure if they found something. I comforted him by letting him know that the only thing that could be found was a slight sign where the colon was damaged, and even that was questionable.

To the doctors' surprise, the X-ray indicated no damage in the lower colon area. They were so baffled by the findings that they decided to do a more complete set of X-rays later, when my father felt stronger.

*

* *

My job was done, and I was ready to leave for home. My father's energy field was fully recovered. The energy centers were of normal size and shape, and the energy was holding between treatments. He was walking about six hundred to eight hundred feet at a time, and the color of his face had nearly returned to normal. Because his energy field was in good condition and holding, Dad was going to be ready to go home in a few days.

The Recovery

My father was sent home two days later. His blood count was normal, and he was walking well. He was released on the condition that he would come back one week later for a full set of abdominal X-rays to try to establish the origin of the bleeding that had occurred earlier.

At the follow-up appointment, the doctors tried all types of diagnostic methods: regular X-ray with and without Barium, CAT scan, and MRI. After seven hours of work, they could not find any sign of internal bleeding or scarring. They did not have any reasonable explanation for their findings.

At home, Dad recovered quite well. Within about a month, he had recovered 97 percent of his breathing capacity. He did not have any more problems with internal bleeding, although no medical treatment had been used to treat that condition.

Part II: What Is This All About?

Healing is often perceived as being unscientific and therefore ineffective. The healer is seen as someone who does not quite fit into society because he or she works outside medical norms. There is a frequently perpetuated false image of healers merely providing comfort to their clients and offering no real medical solutions. Considering that studies indicate that 75 percent of visits to medical doctors are a result of stress [1], healers would provide a very useful service even if they did nothing more than induce a deep sense of relaxation.

To begin, **let me emphasize that I do not advocate using energy healing as a replacement for medical care.** In fact, I require people with whom I am working to be under a doctor's supervision while working with me. Healing is not a cure-all, but it can be a very good supporting tool when combined with medical care. It can provide insights and help in the diagnosis of an illness,[17] lead to adjustments in the dosage of medications, or quickly detect drug sensitivity. For example, I have known people on antibiotics who start having a combination of complaints that do not fit the description

---

[17] Older changes in the energy field show up differently from more recent ones. In chronic illnesses, then, healers can easily pinpoint the origins of the problem, while medical tests have no such capability.

of any specific illness. Despite following the recommended dosages of medication, they feel worse and worse. These people often get better with a single healing session and a change in the type of antibiotic used. The healing session is necessary simply to eliminate the harmful energetic imprint from the field, thus allowing the doctor to determine the exact source of health complaints without being clouded by the unwanted side effects of the antibiotic: allergy to the medication being used or using the wrong type of medication altogether. The results of the session are communicated to the medical doctor, who has the necessary knowledge to change or adjust the medication.

To fully understand healing, one has to practice it. It also requires a completely different frame of reference than that of the exact sciences, which are based on measurements. This makes it difficult to be accepted by the medical establishment, since the only concrete measurements for healing are the results: the person who had a stroke can speak for first time after six months of silence, the improved blood count of a person with leukemia, or the clean X-ray of an untreated bleeding ulcer.

In my practice, I found that the least one can achieve with healing is relaxation, which helps with the regulation of blood pressure, induces a better sleep pattern, and lifts a gloomy mood. These improvements are due to the balancing of the energy field.

In the following pages I will try to answer the most frequently asked questions related to healing.

What are the most important things I learned as a healer?

First, I want people to understand that there is absolutely no difference in energy field make-up that correlates with one's ethnic origin, but there is a very strong correlation with one's attitude toward life. The vibrational frequency of a kindhearted, compassionate person is a delight to work with, while an angry person's field is full of "bumps" resulting from the impeded energy flow related to negative thoughts.

Many people ask me why there are kind people who help everyone but acquire terminal illnesses, while others who are not so nice live a long and healthy life.

The answer I learned through my years of healing is quite interesting. People who focus on others to the extreme often neglect themselves in the process, generating imbalances in their own fields. By the same token, if somebody lives life to the fullest, not getting upset about everyday happenings and recognizing that the ups and down are a normal part of life, their own energy can flow freely, the way it was originally "programmed" at birth.

I also found that the secret of a long and healthy life is balance. Helping other people is commendable and improves one's energy field and health *if it is done with balance*. Enjoying life to the fullest is again a big energy field booster when one finds joy in it (in such a case, the field vibration rate goes up and the colors become brighter), but if it is done to the point of exhaustion, the field is weakened.

I find volunteering and helping others a big boost to the field; in addition to higher vibrational frequency and brighter colors, the field also becomes gentler. But when done in excess, it has a negative effect on the field.

Compassion is an important energy field booster too, but taking over another person's pain just generates pain in us, and no one is helped in the process. The right way of doing it is to find solutions for the other person that are empowering—in other words, do what you can to avoid creating dependence.

If I had to choose only one piece of advice on how to live one's life the healthiest way, I would definitely choose **a balanced mental attitude**. This is no secret, as Hindu yogis have been saying the same thing for the past four millennia. I can see it in a person's field. If somebody practices meditation regularly, the field is much more balanced and the person is more aware when they are doing something unhealthy. This does not necessarily mean that somebody has to meditate for many hours every day, though it's advisable to meditate regularly for at least half an hour each day.

Physical exercise is very good for strengthening the field but does not provide a more balanced approach to life.

An attitude of gratitude is a wonderful energy field booster. The field of a person living in gratitude is gentle, compassionate, has a high vibration, and is a real joy to be around. The presence of such a person makes everybody around him or her feel better. One feels lighter, and the weight of everyday problems no longer seems as daunting.

If you want to have a healthy life:

- Be compassionate to yourself and others

- Meditate, expressing gratitude for all you have

- Exercise in moderation

- Help others while keeping balance regarding your own needs

- Find joy in whatever you are doing, be it your work or taking care of your family

- Eat healthy food and, while eating, think with gratitude about all those (including you) who contributed to bringing that food to your table

I have seen the changes each of the above can produce in the human energy field. Try it!

What is the energy field and how does it work?

Every living or inanimate object has a particular kind of energy field. The field feels like a very low-level current, much like a slight energetic buzzing. The more active fields have a more complex pattern and a stronger feel. The energy field of a stone is very static, having next to no movement, while the field of a plant is quite active. A tree will usually have an active energy field during the summer months and a more subdued one during the winter. The energy field of animals is more complex than that of plants. Generally, the more evolved an animal, the more complex the field.

The healthy field feels even all over the human body. Any disruption of this pattern represents places where healing needs to be applied. The disruptions can be of different types: thickening for pus, heat for pain or inflammation, and local lack of energy for serious internal damage. For example, an acute ulcer feels like ridges of missing energy, while a stroke feels like points of blocked, immobile energy. Also, each illness has a well-defined energy pattern: a certain strain of flu will localize in a certain area of the body and have a distinguishable energy pattern.

In healing, the exact medical diagnosis does not matter. In fact, it is a well-known fact that many sicknesses have the same outward signs. The advantage in healing is that it can find the exact energetic source of a problem, even if medical science does not have a name for it. To a healer, the energy field is like an open book that can be easily read with the palm of one's hand or even just by looking at or thinking about the body.

Certain people can perceive the field through their hands only; others can perceive it only visually, as brighter or darker colors. Some people can sense the field both ways. Brighter colors and an evenly buzzing field indicate a good state of energy balance, which indicates health; darker, dirty colors and energy imbalances indicate sickness. There are well-established esoteric theories about the human energy field. A good review of those can be found in Barbara Brennan's books [2, 3].

The following is what I use as a working model: Every person who has studied biology knows that all our bodily functions are governed by the transmission of signals that are received by the nervous system from the environment or from internal organs. The nervous system, made up of interconnected neurons, responds to these stimuli according to our human physiology, most of which is already in place at birth. Electrical signals are transmitted through some battery-like phenomena that occur at the synapses—the places where two neurons connect. Obviously, if someone knew how to influence the electrical discharges at the synaptic levels, that person could change the overall way the body reacts.

If the neural transmitters are defective, or if the internal organs do not respond in an optimum manner, one can easily imagine *signal attenuations*—that is, the signal level received is not in proportion to the one transmitted, producing a noisy reception, like a radio with static. Anyone who has opened a radio that made crackling noises knows that the way to improve the reception is to dust the components, thereby removing the source of the static. Sometimes a simple brushing is enough; other times, the dirty components need to be washed with alcohol. That is what the healer does: removes the "static"—the energy imbalances—from the field.

What does a healer do during the session?

What the healer does is very similar to the above scenario. A typical session starts with the healer checking the energy field, known as the **aura**, noticing the different types of energy changes. He or she then cleans the debris and repairs the damaged areas by directing energy where necessary.

The healer is only the conduit for the energy used during healing. As strange as it may sound to some, the energy comes from the environment and is directed by the healer using his or her energy field as a conduit. To treat an illness, the healer puts his/her own energy field in the right frequency range, making sure that the person's aura will not be overstressed. A child, an older adult, or a very sick person will be able to take only a lower-energy frequency and amplitude. My researcher friends will probably say that this is preposterous, but I know from my own experience it is true. During healing sessions, I can always feel the energy pouring out of the palms of my hands or from the tips of my fingers. It is a very physical sensation. Sometimes I can even see the energy transferring from my hands into the person's energy field.

Most people have a difficult time accepting the idea of invisible energy fields surrounding our bodies, yet everyone can imagine capturing radio waves from thin air. Just as the electromagnetic waves can be captured by a radio, healing energy can be utilized by a trained person able to capture it. Skilled healers will tell you that the energy they use is not their own.

A good healer will almost always feel more refreshed at the end of a session than at the beginning. There is a good explanation for this. When we direct energy into a person's body using ourselves as a conduit, we are healing ourselves as well. Unfortunately, our sensitivity also makes us pick up all sorts of energetic garbage from our environment: anger, sorrow, or the feelings associated with an illness.

Professor Valerie Hunt did considerable work with energy fields [5, 6]. Her studies document some of the things I have discovered intuitively. Yet, there are still many more questions than answers. I can understand if you as a reader find yourself doubting what is written in these pages. Our mechanistic society does not allow much room for phenomena that can be understood only by using an intuitive frame of reference. That is certainly the case when working with unrepeatable conditions, such as humans who change from one day to the next or even within the boundaries of a single day, and when making judgments based only on results. I myself went through much doubt, and even today I constantly observe my work in search of more answers to my myriad questions as a scientist.

How does the healing session feel from the recipient's point of view?

He or she can usually notice some of the energy changes. The level of sensitivity to the movement of energy is enhanced when the person receiving the healing is relaxed or the illness is in an acute stage. A person who is uptight about the treatment will stop the free flow of energy, very much like shutting off the tap and then waiting for the water to flow. A relaxed person most likely will feel heat when energy is directed into a certain spot or will sense something like a very low-grade electric current during energy rebalancing. In rare cases, such as when a person is very sensitive or when the illness is severe, like a broken bone, a low level of pain might be felt due to the intense energy exchange.

What is the correspondence between the physical body and the energy centers?

It is very interesting for a healer to look at a chiropractic chart that lists the nervous plexi as they correspond to **chakras**, the seven main energy centers used by healers. The base chakra is located at the coccygeal plexus area; the second in the sacral plexus area; the third in the solar plexus area; the fourth in the cardiac plexus area; the fifth in the cervical plexus/thyroid area; the sixth in the pituitary gland area, which is located deep inside the brain; and the seventh in the pineal gland area, also located inside the brain. This leads me to believe that ancient doctors could feel these centers even before science started documenting them through dissection.

Can anyone be a healer?

Yes. I believe that anyone who has an honest concern for the welfare of others and is willing to devote the necessary time and effort to learn how to do it can achieve a good level of proficiency. Of course, some people have a special talent for healing or are even born with the intuitive knowledge about how to do it, very similar to young prodigies in any field. Healing is very much like playing a musical instrument: if someone really has his/her heart into it, he/she will be able to do it well and will continuously improve with practice.

What conditions must be met to be an effective healer?

A healer must deeply care for people and not be attached to the result. The latter might sound strange, but it is very important. If the healer is attached to the outcome, he or she will have a hard time letting go of the client receiving the healing sessions when it is obvious that energy healing is not the best option—and sometimes it isn't. A ruptured appendix, for example, should be treated with emergency surgery. However, even on the trip to the hospital, a healer can help control the pain and damage.

A good healer should also recognize his or her own limitations. For example, emotional pain is fairly easy to detect and treat with healing, but if somebody is mentally imbalanced, deeply depressive, or has a high potential for violence, it is imperative to refer that person to the appropriate health-care professional. In this latter case, the healer can step in (under the doctor's supervision) to help the person be more responsive to the medication as healing enables a more effective processing of drugs.

Just as medical science does not have solutions for all illnesses, neither does energy healing. Considering that healers have no official status in our society and that they cannot guarantee a cure, they should never assume the role of a main health-care professional.

Does the recipient have to believe in healing?

Despite what some may think, the recipient does *not* have to believe in healing for it to be effective. Of course, if the person expects success, very much like in cases treated by medical doctors with traditional medications or treatments, he/she will have a faster recovery.

Years ago, I worked with the mother of one of my friends. The lady was quite impressive, one of the first feminists to receive the Order of Canada for her work. She had great difficulty accepting the idea that such a gentle healing treatment could work on her Parkinson's disease when medical science had not been effective. She greeted me every time with, "Here comes hocus-pocus again." However, after about five sessions she was able to move around in her home without falling down repeatedly. After a few more sessions, she started recognizing people, went out of the house for the first time in two years, was able to walk in and out of stores using her walker, and started to cook again. Nevertheless, she never told me that she accepted healing as being real.

How does energy work compare with other methods of healing?

Once I had the very special opportunity to compare medical, chiropractic, and healing diagnoses. The medical doctor knew from the patient's complaints that the knees were damaged by sports activities, and the doctor could make an evaluation of what might be wrong. The chiropractor checked the patient and was able to provide more details regarding the muscles involved. I was able to define which one of the knees was worse. This latter fact was confirmed by the chiropractor after a more detailed evaluation. All three of us worked on that person. The doctor prescribed some anti-inflammatory medication. The chiropractor did bone and muscle manipulation. My energy work reduced the pain and improved the overall mobility level. Each practitioner did something to help the person in different ways.

When does an illness appear in the energy field and how long does it stay?

Every sickness first appears as a disturbance in the energy field long before the person feels ill. If someone has regular energy checkups, he or she has a good chance of staying healthy. An interesting phenomenon that I repeatedly witnessed in my practice is that people with long-lasting degenerative diseases get healed from an energetic point of view and feel perfectly well, but their medical tests take some time to catch up. This indicates that the energy field, not the physical body, governs our health. Perhaps this has something to do with the long-held belief that we are composed of mind, body, and soul.

Sooner or later, all healers notice another intriguing phenomenon: the energy field holds memories long lost from the conscious mind.[18] I know people who lost a loved one ten years earlier and who still have painful memories stored in the energy field above the heart chakra. These memories can cause unexplained health problems, but once they are removed from the energy field, the person feels much better. I have also found childhood injuries that were more than forty years old. Most people did not even remember being injured, yet the energetic disturbances were still lodged in the field above the place where a bone was broken before. These people invariably told me that they remembered the injury after the healing session. Maybe it is part of the mechanics of the body releasing the trauma at a physical level.

What about the soul?

Healers can see when a person is ready to depart. There is a very clear energetic sign: the field starts gradually

---

[18] This was confirmed by Candace Pert's work published in 1997 [10].

disappearing from the legs as if it is going to leave through the top of the head. Where does that energy go? Is that what happens with people in near-death experiences?

The only reasonable explanation I found was in the yogic tradition. Yoga believes that the soul can travel out of the body and return as long as the etheric "silver cord" connecting the soul to the physical body is not broken. Once that is broken, there will be no return.

What are some representative cases?

To begin, I need to mention that every energy field with which I ever worked had a slightly different combination of pattern and frequency. As such, every healing session is different, and the healing process proceeds in ways particular to the specific imbalance/illness.

As discussed earlier, a good healer is sometimes capable of detecting the sources of an illness when medical science cannot find a cause due to technological limitations. Years ago, one of my uncles had severe pains up and down his right leg that extended into his back. The doctors did not know how to help him. Novocain injections in his back relieved the pain, but only for a limited time. This went on for eight months before I found out about it and performed an energy scan on his back and leg. I found that he had injured his knee internally, damaging the meniscus. I suggested that he ask the doctor for an X-ray that could detect such an injury. The X-ray confirmed the energetic findings.

In another case, a young friend had been diagnosed with epilepsy and was having frequent *grand mal*[19] seizures despite the medication prescribed for his condition. The doctors could not find the source of the problem. The situation seemed hopeless. Upon examining the energy field, I found that his skull bone was chipped at the back of his head. The energy was missing, as if someone had drilled a hole through it. I felt the injury was an old one, probably from his childhood. When I questioned him about it, he confirmed that he had experienced a bad head injury as a child. He never considered the old injury as a possible source of his problem because the doctors never mentioned it. Once the energy damage was repaired, his seizures stopped.

There were other interesting cases. One of them was that of an uncle who had a stroke; six months later he still could not speak any of the four languages that he knew well. For six months he could utter no more than "yes" in his mother tongue. After a local scan of the head,

---

[19] Epilepsy is a condition caused by abnormal electrical discharges in the brain. *grand al* is the most serious kind of epileptic seizure; it causes the person to fall to the ground, twitch, and foam at the mouth. The *grand mal* is followed by a deep sleep or trance-like condition. The *petit mal* is the less intense form of epileptic seizure; for brief periods, the person seems to be in a world of his own.

I found the place of the blockage: the energy was not moving through an area smaller than the size of a dime. My uncle started talking again the day after the area of the energetic blockage was cleaned. According to his family, after the fifth session, he regained a vocabulary rich with words he had not used for twenty years. Was it instant remission? It was a bit too much of a coincidence to be only that!

Another case worth mentioning is the case of a person who had congestive heart failure. He came to me looking very haggard. His face was very pale, he was retaining water, and he could walk only short distances before becoming tired. This is a condition considered by the medical sciences as untreatable, with "instant remissions" sometimes happening for no tangible reason. The energy field in his heart area looked like a volcanic crater; electric sparks were coming out of an opening the size of a melon. At the base of the skull I could feel an energy rush trying to make up for the tired

ness. The energy in the legs was stagnated, and the kidney area was obviously in distress, holding a lot of accumulated energy. The most unusual part was finding an under-functioning pineal region. After a few sessions he was able to run up two flights of stairs without any problems.

Another case that raised many unsettling questions was that of a cancer-related amputee who was still experiencing shock pains twenty years after the surgery. These pains were unbearable and could not be helped with medication. During the energetic scan I could still find the cancer pain lodged in the former knee, shin bone, and ankle area, even though the leg had been severed above the knee. The most unsettling finding in this case was that the energy field was complete, as if the whole leg was still there. This raises the question of how the nervous system preserves the memory of periodic pain twenty years later and, more importantly, whether we are primarily energy or physical beings.

The person stopped having the shooting pains after the cancer pattern was removed from the field.

Is there a special time when healing is more effective?

Typically, it is easiest to correct an energy imbalance immediately after it occurs. This phenomenon is well known to doctors who can more easily treat an acute rather than a chronic illness. From an energetic point of view, the difference between acute and chronic is very noticeable. An acute illness can be remedied quite easily, while chronic illness feels like major damage to the system, involving not only the area known to be affected but other areas as well.

Is healing always successful?

Healing may not always be successful. When a person has a vested interest in staying sick, there is nothing healing alone can do to completely resolve the problem. The case of a person with Grave's disease comes to my mind. He came to me with a thyroid as large as the front of his neck that protruded over the sides of his neck. His eyes were bulging considerably, showing a very advanced form of the disease. After the second session, his eyes looked normal and the thyroid was one-third smaller in height and half its original width. The medical tests, according to him, confirmed an unexpected improvement, with the thyroid ten times less active.

When asked if he was happy with the developments, he said, "I do not know what I am going to do if I get any better. I hardly have time now to do all the things I wish to do. How am I going to do all those things when I am healthy and must return to work?" Although I urged him to envision his life after recovery, he refused, citing various excuses.

His thyroid function stopped improving, and tests one month later showed the same hormone levels as before. As the old saying goes, "Watch out what you wish for, as you might get it." As I found out later, in such cases one must apply a combination of healing and hypnotherapy. The person must be regressed to the original source of illness and healed at that point in time. But this is a topic large enough for another book.

*

*   *

The energetic models and case studies presented above are my own. Other healers have very similar experiences. I trust that the multifaceted way in which I tried to present this information will give some readers the courage to experience for themselves the marvelous results of healing. I also hope that some medical researchers will be motivated enough by these experiences to delve into this field.

Part III: Playing with Energy

Every time I make a presentation, people ask me if there is any way they could feel the energy field. As the only way to convince somebody that they can truly feel energy is to provide a way to access it, I decided to add to this new edition of the book some exercises, some that can be done alone and some requiring a partner.

Exercises that can be done alone

1. Dim the lights in the room. I find it best to switch off all lights and then light a candle, positioning it behind you so it provides an indirect light. Rub your palms together for one to two minutes then put your hands together as shown in Figure A below.

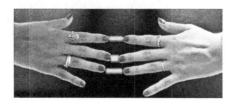

Figure A: Seeing the energy field between the fingers.

Slowly move your hands apart about half an inch (one centimeter). You will see a haze between your fingers that is the energy field. To improve your chances of seeing the energy, slowly move your hands closer then farther apart, since different people have different energy field strengths.

2. Rub your hands together for one to two minutes then move your hands apart as if you have a balloon between your hands (see Figure B). Slowly move your hands closer and then farther apart. At some point you will encounter some slight resistance, which is the energy field.

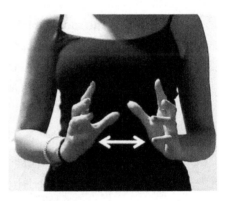

Figure B: Feeling the energy field between your hands.

Exercises requiring a partner

1. Dim the lights and hang a dark sheet on the wall. Ask your partner to sit or stand with his/her back to the wall, about one foot (thirty centimeters) away from the wall. Ask your partner to take ten deep breaths then look in the direction of your partner's head and shoulder area, focusing a few inches past your partner. You should see a light haze around your partner's shoulder/head area, where the field is usually strongest (see Figure C).

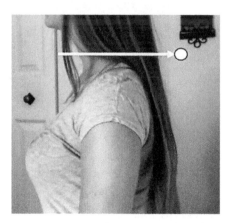

Figure C: Seeing the energy field around the head and shoulders. The dot shows where to focus your eyes.

2. Ask your partner to take off his/her shoes and walk a bit, noticing how his/her legs feel.

Slightly bend your fingers (see Figure D) and slowly move your hands about an inch (two centimeters) away from one of the legs, as if combing the energy field downward. Comb the field **of one leg only** twenty times then ask your partner to walk. The leg you just worked on should feel lighter than the other.

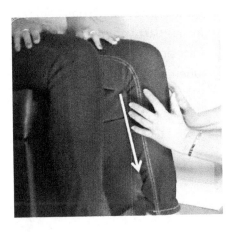

Figure D: "Combing" the energy field.

Make sure to comb the energy on the other leg too then ask your partner to check again how it feels to walk.

3. This is a more advanced exercise. Next time a family member complains about problems breathing due to the flu, slowly comb the field (about two inches off the body) above the lung twenty times in front of the body above the lung

area and twenty times in the back (see Figure E). As you comb, visualize in your mind that you are removing the inflammation. The person should breathe much easier after that.

<u>Make sure to wash your hands under running water (no soap required) after the combing exercises to remove any energy patterns you might have picked up!</u>

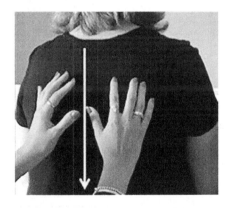

Figure E: Cleaning the energy field of the person with flu. Do the same on the front of the body.

Part IV: Final Thoughts

I started on the healing path at a loss to explain what I was doing and having practically no one with whom to share my experiences. I felt very much alone as I tried to hide my healing capabilities, which kept coming up every time I saw somebody in need. It was very hard to know that I could probably aid a person's healing, but at the same time realizing they would probably not accept my offer—or, even worse, that they would ridicule me.

Over the years I read a lot and took healing courses in traditional Hindu, Japanese, and Chinese techniques, as well as Healing Touch and Clinical Hypnosis. I knew after a while that I was not as "crazy" as I thought I was in the beginning, but I was still afraid to openly talk about it.

With the passing of years, I found that doing healing work ceased to be a choice. I could no longer get away from it. It had become a part of me, and I felt grateful every time I could help the healing process in a person. In time I had the opportunity to experience all types of energy imbalances, from the common cold to stroke, asthma, back pain, cancer, and broken bones. Each case was and still is a voyage of discovery and a wonderful experience through the stories told by the energy field. I am continuously amazed how such a gentle treatment can accomplish so much in such a short time.

The fact that my father was helped by healing was a precious gift for all of us. He lived another eight months, a time during which he continued to be active: traveling, helping others, and enjoying his family. Unfortunately, he felt and looked so good that even his doctor did not believe him when Dad started once again having discomfort due to a new cancer, this time induced by the experimental radiation therapy applied after the lung surgery. By the time he got to the hospital, it was too late, and healing could only help control his pain.

Four days before he passed away, Dad, a very enthusiastic engineer all his life, asked me to explain to him something that was part of my engineering profession: how integrated chips—which made possible today's iPads and notebooks—were designed and manufactured. Too weak to listen to my explanation, he told me we would have to finish the discussion some other time. I was heartbroken. I knew by then that there could be no "other time." But he kept his date. One night, shortly after his passing, I found myself again in my dreams in the place where everything is made of bright, shimmering light. Dad came to me, and we sat down on a bench and had a lengthy discussion about chip technologies, very much as we would if he were still alive.

At the end, we discussed how the family was taking his departure. I told him how much Andrei, my son, and I missed his gentle bear hugs. As we finished our discussion, he stood up and gave me a big hug. The feeling was so physically real I woke up and cried for a long time. I still missed my father terribly, but his hug gave me the feeling that Dad was still with us in some way.

I wanted to write this book since that night in the hospital room when I had to decide between keeping my promise to my mother or using my healing techniques to help my father. Only after Dad's passing did I finally find the time to write it. I know my father would have been happy with the results of this book, as it helped my Mom understand and accept what I was doing. After reading the book, both she and my sister started taking advantage of my healing capabilities and knowledge.

Bibliography

[1] Borysenko, Joan, Ph.D. *Guilt Is the Teacher, Love Is the Lesson,* Warner Books, 1990, ISBN 0-446- 39224-3, 43.

[2] Brennan, Barbara. *Hands of Light,* Bantam Books, 1988, ISBN 0-553-34539-7.

[3] Brennan, Barbara. *Light Emerging,* Bantam Books, 1993, ISBN 0-553-35456-6.

[4] Hartzell Bro, Harmon: *A Seer Out of Season—The Life of Edgar Cayce,* A Signet Book, 1989, ISBN 0-451-16479-2.

[5] Hunt, Valerie, Prof., Dr.: *Infinite Mind,* Malibu Publishing Company, 1995, ISBN 0-9643988-0-x.

[6] Hunt, Valerie, Prof., Dr.: *The Human Energy Field and Health* (videotape), Bioenergy Fields Foundation, 1993.

[7] Karp, Reba Ann: *Edgar Cayce Encyclopedia of Healing,* Warner Books, 1986, ISBN 0-446-30981-8.

[8] Kilner, Waiter, J., B.A., M.B., etc.: *The Aura,* Samuel Weiser, New York, 1978, ISBN 0-87728- 215-3.

[9] Leadbetter, C. W.: *The Chakras,* The Theosophical Publishing House, Wheaton, Illinois, U.S.A./Madras, India/London, England.

[10] Pert, Candace, Ph.D.: *Molecules of Emotion*, Scribner, ISBN-10: 0-684-84634-9.

Acknowledgments

First and foremost, my deepest thanks go to my teacher, Mary Ann Geoffrey, who taught me a lot about how to be an ethical healer and guided my steps, read my books, and offered support whenever I needed it. Thanks also go to her husband, Steve Geoffrey, who was kind enough to read this book and offer his input, encouraging me in my endeavor of bringing it to life.

I am also indebted to the doctors who were open-minded and agreed to work with me: David Brownstein, Jeffrey Nussbaum, Richard Ng, Al Scarchilli, and Paul Parente. They helped me trust my talents by accepting my input on cases that had no solutions in traditional medicine at a time when such an attitude was considered medical heresy.

I also thank all the people with whom I worked and who taught me so much about resilience and open-mindedness. Their energy fields showed me the most wonderful stories of healing.

The support of my friends and family who helped me bring this book to life is greatly appreciated: Renata Stoica, Andrei Stoica, Ecaterina Gerson, Kelly and Dakota

Bruce, Tsila and Rachael Pleasant, Michelle Michael, and Laura Molina.

I am also lucky to have a son who never wavered in his belief that one day I will be able to fully take advantage of my healing talents and share them with people worldwide!

Last, but not least, thank you, my reader! If you liked my book, please take the time and write a review to help those who need to decide whether this book is for them.

About the Author

Susana Stoica, a Ph.D. in computer engineering, is an inventor, healer, writer, and speaker/teacher. She practiced her engineering profession on three continents, which gave her an appreciation of the unique and common cultural and healing traditions of people from different parts of the world.

Susana is a Healing Touch Practitioner, Hypnotherapist, and Journey Practitioner and is self-taught in many other alternative healing methods. She strives continuously to gain ever deeper insights into the workings of the human energy system and its relationship with the physical body, being amazed and humbled by its complexity and perfect functionality. She lives in Michigan in the United States.

Made in the USA
Las Vegas, NV
07 January 2023

65200155R00066